Dieting For Hair Growth Manual

Using Food To Grow Long & Healthy Strong Hair

AUTHOR BREANNA RUTTER

TABLE OF CONTENTS

INTRODUCTION TO
DIETING FOR HAIR GROWTH
MANUAL

"The Dieting For Hair Growth Manual is a pocket guide that will enhance your hair growth through means of eating foods that specifically aid the growth of your hair. We will talk about foods that promote a healthy body with hair growth being one of many desirable byproducts. There are a variety of reasons why someone wants to grow longer hair whether they are recovering from hair loss, thinning hair, or maybe even for just cosmetic appeal. No matter the health condition or type of hair you have, the suggestions given in this manual will grow anyone's hair to longer lengths by simply using specific vitamins, minerals, and nutrients that directly aid the growth of hair!

Dieting for hair growth will only work if you eat the foods that are best for hair growth while also eating foods that will nourish your body as given in the Chapter 7 title "Dieting For Hair Growth". As highlighted in this chapter, you will understand the fundamental elements you have to have in your diet such as; B Vitamins, Omega Fats, and Alkaline Foods so that you can ensure the most hair growth from the foods you are eating.

This manual breaks down vitamins, nutrients and minerals that are essential for contributing to the growth of your hair. You will be supplied with simple easy to follow growth oil recipes, a hair care regimen, supplement suggestions and much more.

Please enjoy this informative read and apply everything taught in this book on a consistent basis to grow your hair!"
Sincerely Breanna

1 THE HAIR GROWTH CYCLE

Understanding the life cycle of hair will give you the basic foundation of knowing how long it should take to see results from your hair growth efforts. Knowing the behavioral characteristics of hair growth will indicate whether or not your diet is improving the results of your hair and if the shedding you are experiencing is normal. The hair growth cycle will help you to know how long you should expect to see results with your hair to make sure that the things you are doing are really making a difference!

Hair encounters three stages within its growth cycle. Each individual hair you are growing on your head can be in different stages of its life cycle and because of that, you lose on average 80 to 100 strands of hair daily. Given that you have about 100,000 strands of hair on your head in total, don't be alarmed about shedding that many strands because this is a normal process that has to take place. If you think about it, shedding makes up way less than 1% of hair that you have on your scalp right now! Now let's discuss the life cycle of hair.

The Anagen Phase is the 1st phase of the hair life cycle as this is the growing phase because a new hair has begun growing. Since all of your hair is not in the Anagen Phase at once, it will take time before you will notice thickness because other hairs have to enter this phase as well. This phase lasts 2 to 6 years.

The Catagen Phase is the 2nd phase in which your hair is transitioning towards the Telogen phase. The hair is separating from your follicle (see definition guide) and moving upward towards your pore, or the surface of your scalp to fall out as shed hair. This phase lasts 1 to 2 weeks.

The Telogen Phase is the 3rd phase in which the hair is resting because the dermal papilla (see definition guide) separates from the follicle and then moves upward to begin growing a brand new hair. This phase lasts 2 to 4 months.

It is important that you completely understand the hair growth cycle so that you can gauge how long it should take for your hair to show signs of growth! The Telogen Phase and the Anagen Phase are the only two phases that allows you to see growth in hair even though the Anagen Phase alone is the cycle that yields growth. The time frames between these two phases are 2 months to 6 years. You should not have to wait 6 years to see your growth efforts because remember, all hair is not in the same phase at the same time!

The golden time frame to stick with when trying specific things to gain significant hair growth will take no longer than 2 to 4 months. You should see growth in as little as 2 months and if you do not see growth, 4 months is the longest time you will need to wait to see results of growth.

If you have remained consistent in trying a specific recommendation or diet plan as instructed for growing your hair, and you see no signs of growth within 2 to 4 months, go ahead and try another recommendation until you find success with growing back the edges of your hair!

2 UNDERSTANDING HAIR PH

Have you ever experienced difficulty maintaining smooth hair because of dryness and constant flyways while trying to maintain smooth hair? What about frizzy hair? Frizzy hair will ruin any hairstyle and the common situations that cause frizziness are moments when your hair is either straight or in braids or twists. The reason why frizzy or dry hair is hard to beat is because the hair is not PH balanced! PH balance has a lot to do with the health and behavior of your hair to achieve certain results. In relation to growing out your hair, your hair is left prone to breakage if it is not in its ideal range of PH!

The PH scale measures how acidic or alkaline a solution is and the scale ranges from 1 (acidic) to 14 (alkaline). Water has a PH of 7 (neutral) and is used to compare the acidity or alkalinity of a solution. The ideal PH range of hair is 4.5 to 5.5. Use PH balanced products especially if you want to achieve your most healthy hair! The reason why is because when your hair is in contact with an acidic product, it will cause your cuticles (refer to definition guide) to flatten resulting in smooth & healthy moisturized strands of hair. Hair in contact with an alkaline solution causes the cuticles to raise & swell resulting in rough & frizzy dry hair.

To grow your hair, it is high priority to always keep your hair in the range of 4.5 to 5.5 and a great way to do this, is to make sure that your hair care products are PH balanced. If you do not know the PH of your hair care products, test your products with Litmus Strips. You can find these strips in specialty stores and online. If you want products that are already PH balanced, I highly suggest HowToBlackHair.com referred hair care products specifically formulated for maintaining healthy hair.

3 B VITAMINS

The vitamins most responsible for increasing hair growth are B Vitamins! Having a balanced healthy diet allows for you to receive a balance of B Vitamins naturally and if your food choices are not rich in supplying wide range of B Vitamins, supplementing will be key for increasing your hair growth. In a future chapter, you will be supplied with a list of foods that have naturally occurring high levels of B Vitamins (Chapter 6) along with other vitamins and nutrients as well but before moving on to the list of foods, it's important to know what B Vitamins are responsible for when increasing the growth of your hair.

There are 8 different kinds of B Vitamins required for health such as; B1, B2, B3, B5, B6, B7, B9 and B12. Supplementing for Complex B Vitamins gives you adequate vitamin dosage most healthy for your body and this helps because it takes the guesswork away from how much of a certain kind of food you must eat! Supplementing is an option of course while it is suggested instead to seek B Vitamins through your food choices since vitamin absorption work best because vitamins depend on other vitamins to help your small intestine absorb them.

The B Vitamins that contribute specifically to increased hair growth are; B6, B7 (biotin), and B12. The superior B Vitamin of them all, even though all of them are essential for hair growth, is B7 or commonly referred to as Biotin. Unlike other B Vitamins, B7 has to be taken daily because your liver does not hold storage of this vitamin, it constantly passes from your body every time you urinate. Adults (19 years +) can take at least 30 mg of B7 daily and if you choose to take a B Complex instead, dosage in this case is no more than 50mg daily.

4 OMEGA FATS

Omega Fats never come up in conversation when speaking about healthy hair dieting and/or hair pills! In chapter seven titled, "Hair Vitamins", we will enlighten you about hair pills to let you discern whether they are worth the hype or not but for now, we will focus on Omega Fats!

There are three different kinds of Omega Fats that are essential for good health and they are; Omega 3, Omega 6 and Omega 9. Explaining why they are named the way they are veers into the scientifical side, and its best to just know how they actually benefit your hair growth rather than just knowing the way their elements are fixated within an atom.

All Omega Fats improves blood circulation as well as internally moisturizes your hair and scalp. Regulated blood pressure creates healthy skin which normalizes skin shedding, dandruff issues and moisture levels. Their benefits also allows your hair and scalp (skin in general) to retain adequate levels of water which will improve hair and skin elasticity. All Omega Fats reverse hair loss and dry scalp to lessen any present skin conditions such as eczema or psoriasis for example. Lacking a healthy amount of Omega Fats in your diet will cause you to crave fatty foods (like deep fried foods for example).

Since our bodies use Omega 3 ,6 and unsaturated fats to create Omega 9, it is important that we receive enough Omega 3 and 6 in our diet since our body can create Omega 9 Fat. Let's dig a little bit deeper to understand specifically, what each of the Omega Fats are responsible for in regards to hair growth!

Omega 3 Fat is abundantly obtained through fish, nuts, and plant based oils (in that order). Since Omega 3 Fat cannot naturally produce within the body, it is an essential fat while Omega 9 is a non-essential fat (since our bodies can easily create this specific fatty acid). Omega 3 slows down both forms of Alopecia, Traction Alopecia and Areata Alopecia. For more information on alopecia and how to specifically treat it, refer to the book titled, How To Reverse Traction Alopecia Manual. Omega 3 slows hair loss for those who are thinning or losing hair due to genetics, it also prevents hair loss due to a diet lacking in vitamins, nutrients, minerals, and stimulates your sebaceous gland to increase sebum production (refer to definition guide). Adults are suggested to not exceed 4000 mg dosage of Omega 3 Fat and to consult with a doctor before consuming by supplementation.

Omega 6 Fat is abundantly obtained through poultry and plant based oils (in that order). Omega 6 Fat also cannot naturally produce within our bodies, which classifies it as an essential fat. Omega 6 Fat also lessens the progression of various skin conditions. This Omega Fat is king when it comes to maintaining moisturized hair and a moisturized scalp. Adults are suggested to not exceed 7 to 16 grams daily of Omega 6 Fat and if you take blood thinners, consult with your primary physician on your consumption of Omega 6 Fat.

Omega 9 is abundantly obtained from vegetables oils with the highest percentage of Omega 9 Fat in safflower, olive and canola oil (in that order). This fat improves your immunity and contributes to a small degree towards the pliability of your hair. This fatty acid (omega oil) is created within your body from Omega 3 and 6 Fats so that is why this oil should consumed sparingly due in part that it is mostly a saturated fat which is bad for your heart health.

5 THICKENING FINE HAIR

Thickening fine hair can be done from the inside and from the outside which requires your discipline to eat in terms for thicker hair and to apply hair thickening oil treatments to your hair on a daily basis. A combination of both inward and outward treatments will get you closer to thicker hair a lot faster than just choosing to take one or the other independently. Please note that if you are naturally born with fine hair or thin hair, your thickening efforts are only in appearance, you cannot thicken your hair permanently but you can restore thicker hair if your thick hair started to thin!

Thick Hair: your ponytail width, with all of your hair gathered, is the width of a quarter or larger

Thin Hair: your ponytail width, with all of your hair gathered, is the width of a nickel or smaller

Fine Hair: your individual strands of hair are smaller in size (diameter) to regular sewing thread

Zinc (mineral) and L-Cysteine (an amino acid) are most effective for thickening your hair. L-Cysteine is a sulfur containing amino acid easily found in protein rich foods such as chicken, turkey, milk and eggs and also in broccoli. This amino acid passes through your blood stream, detoxifies your scalp and allows the diameter of your hair to increase in circumference. Zinc is abundant in red meats, pumpkin seeds, shrimp, and soy products as well. Zinc creates healthier cells and aids the assimilation of protein to lessen shedding which encourages thicker stronger hair. Consult with your doctor if you want to increase your levels of zinc safely and also, try out these recommended hair thickening oil recipes!

When choosing essential oils and carrier oils to thicken thin hair, your oils must possess unique qualities such as the ability to retain or add protein to thicken hair that is fine no matter if your hair is thick or thin. Refer to the definition guide to understand the differences between these types of hair!

ESSENTIAL OILS TO THICKEN HAIR
Lavender and Ylang Ylang Essential Oil

CARRIER OILS TO THICKEN HAIR
Castor, Coconut, Jamaican Black Castor and
Grass Fed Oil

OIL RECIPES TO THICKEN HAIR

(Recipes are created based on how well the scents complement one another)

Lavender Oil Blend

6 drops of Lavender Essential Oil
1 tbsp. of Castor Oil
1 tbsp. of Coconut Oil

Ylang Ylang Oil Blend

6 drops of Ylang Ylang Essential Oil
1 ounce (2 tbsp.) of Grass Fed Butter

(Jamaican Black Castor Oil can be used alone!)

6 DIETING FOR HAIR GROWTH

Hair growth from healthy eating is a natural byproduct of a diet high in nutrients, minerals, and vitamins! Dieting for hair growth encourages you to actually eat better which in turn, directly benefits your state of health even though you are seeking a diet specific to growing your hair! Diets usually last as long as you are willing to accept restrictions so opt instead for food choices that you actually enjoy so that eating them doesn't become a chore. The problem with dieting or only eating specific foods for hair growth, is that it can put you in the position of ignoring foods that you actually enjoy, even if they don't yield the highest percentage of a specific vitamin, mineral, or nutrient! That is why a list of extremely healthy foods (alkaline foods) will be suggested to give you a wide range of food options to eat. Alkaline foods purify your body allowing you to have healthier hair and scalp. Acidic foods affect your hair poorly since any nutrients, minerals and vitamins from these foods are first distributed to your organs before reaching less important areas such as your hair and skin. The key to eating for hair growth is to constantly rotate your specific selection of foods and more importantly, flavor them in different ways to taste so that you aren't becoming annoyed because you have to eat certain foods.

Before planning your new diet for hair growth, it's important to know what foods contain the vitamins, minerals and nutrients responsible for actually growing your hair of course! Previously we discussed the importance B Vitamins and Omega Fats play into growing your hair and to help you yield your best results, you will be equipped with a list of the highest occurring Omega Fats, vitamins, and nutrients for your growing efforts! Following next, are food suggestions that contain the highest amounts of vitamins, nutrients, and minerals!

VITAMINS & NUTRIENTS
FOR HAIR GROWTH

Omega 3 Fatty Acid – improves scalp blood circulation
Omega 6 Fatty Acid – controls eczema and scalp conditions
Omega 9 Fatty Acid – increases hair elasticity
Vitamin B12 – oxygenates blood vessels of hair shaft base
Vitamin B7 (Biotin or Vitamin H) – reverses hair loss
Vitamin B6 – stops DHT production which thins hair

FOODS HIGH IN HAIR GROWTH
VITAMINS AND NUTRIENTS

OMEGA 3	OMEGA 6	OMEGA 9
Flax Seeds 133% Walnuts 113% Sardines 61% Flaxseed Oil 57%	Brazil Nuts 377% Sunflower Seeds 473% Pine Nuts 32%	Safflower Oil 77% Olive Oil 75% Peanut Oil 48%
VITAMIN B12	VITAMIN B7	VITAMIN B6
Clams 1041% Beef Liver 1178% Bran Cereal 300% Mackerel 269%	Peanuts 88% Almonds 49% Sweet Potato 29% Egg Yolk 27%	Sunflower Seeds 94% Salmon 40% Banana 41%

% = percentage of nutritional value per serving based on
the requirements of a 2,000 calorie diet

Eating alkaline foods is the most natural way to supply your body with high levels of vitamins, nutrients, and minerals without the need of supplementing since these foods offer a wide array of everything essential for a healthy diet. Use the recommended list of foods below to aid your diet for hair growth. To know how many servings and calories are required for you, research to find out your caloric needs as this is uniquely based on your age, gender, height and weight. Consume the highest rated foods frequently for your best growth results! Rate is based on highest nutritional value and alkalinity!

ALKALINE FOODS		
1ST RATE ALKALINE FOODS	2ND RATE ALKALINE FOODS	3ND RATE ALKALINE FOODS
Raw Spinach	Olive Oil	Apples
Raw Broccoli	Green Tea	Almonds
Artichoke	Raw Zucchini	Avocados
Brussel Sprouts	Sweet Potato	Tomatoes
Red Cabbage	Raw Peas	Fresh Corn
Raw Celery	Sprouted Grains	Mushrooms
Cauliflower	Raw Eggplant	Turnip Greens
Carrots	Alfalfa Sprouts	Olives
Potato Skin	Raw Green Beans	Soybeans
Alfalfa Grass	Beets	Bell Peppers
Cucumber	Blueberries	Radish
Collards	Pears & Mangoes	Pineapple
Seaweed	Papayas	Cherries
Onion	Figs & Dates	Wild Rice
Asparagus	Tangerines	Strawberries
Lemon & Lime	Melon	Apricot

7 HAIR GROWTH VITAMINS

Hair growth vitamins have always been a part of the hair growth conversation and we are only in the beginning of this growing debate and craze! The demand for hair pills are increasingly growing in popularity due to many celebrity endorsements who swear by them for growth. Hair pills work and don't work depending on the each individual's experience and this chapter is to help you understand hair pills and how well they contribute to hair growth. This chapter will help you discern whether or not hair pills are worth the hype or not!

Hair pills help improve the health of your hair if you are having a difficult time receiving adequate supply of vitamins, nutrients, and minerals. This is understandable for many individuals who have zero access to healthy foods whether for financial reasons or availability of those foods. The flip side to this also, is that some people can eat better if they choose to sacrifice bad foods for good foods. If you can afford to improve your diet in any way, even if that means all you can afford is a bag of apples or a bunch of greens, do the best you can! Not only will your body thank you but your hair will also have a chance to thrive to its highest potential!

Hair growth vitamins are nothing more than a multivitamin with ingredients focused more heavily on B Vitamins as well as other nutrients and minerals highlighted in this manual. Hair growth vitamins may not work well for those with poor diets being that your vital organs will take advantage of the vitamin before your hair can become affected. Hair growth vitamins can and will work, but a healthy balanced diet is ultimately best for hair growth.

8 REVERSE THINNING HAIR

To reverse thinning hair, you can also focus on using hair products that are formulated to encourage thicker hair. Refer to the book, How To Fix Thinning Hair Manual, to solely focus on successfully reversing your thin or thinning hair. There are a variety of reasons that could have caused your hair to thin such as; health issues, aggressive styling, or a natural progression of thinning from aging. Growing back thicker hair is possible and your process to doing so will include a wide array of solutions that range from topical thickening treatments, hairstyling, maintenance habits, and even the option to go the surgical route if you so choose! Understanding how to revert thinning hair can be quite challenging especially when patience comes into play because it is required to wait a period of time in conjunction with the natural growth cycle of your hair to allow yourself time to recover and see results.

This manual focuses on growing back thicker hair in simple easy steps involving growth treatments, hair care regimens and the option of dieting specifically for thickness and so much more! The skills required to achieve thicker hair are of a minimum skill level paired with a vast array of hair knowledge so that you can understand why you have to do certain things to your hair, to maintain and encourage the health of it. This manual will thoroughly educate you about your hair as well as provide a multitude of solutions that will help you to grow your hair thick and healthy.

To give you an idea of some of the information that will be given in the book, you will be able to use some of the Hair Oil Recipes right now that are only exclusively given in the How To Fix Thinning Hair Manual!

OIL RECIPES TO THICKEN YOUR HAIR

(Recipes are created based on how well the scents complement one another)(For the highest nutritional quality of oil, choose Unrefined Cold Pressed Virgin Oils)

Lavender Oil Blend
(For Thickness)

6 drops of Lavender Essential Oil
1 tbsp. of Castor Oil
1 tbsp. of Coconut Oil

Ylang Ylang Oil Blend
(Thickness + Strength)

6 drops of Ylang Ylang Essential Oil
1 ounce (2 tbsp.) of Grass Fed Butter Oil

Jamaican Black Castor Oil
(Thickness + Strength)

1 ounce (2 tbsp.) of Jamaican Black Castor Oil

Bay Oil Blend
(For Stronger Hair)

6 drops of Bay Essential Oil
1 tbsp. of Argan Oil
1 tbsp. of Avocado Oil

THICKENING OIL APPLICATION + REGIMEN

THIS CAN BE DONE DAILY!

Step #1 Use an applicator bottle to apply thin lines of Thickening Hair Oil Recipe onto your scalp.

Step #2 Message scalp with the pads of your fingers for about 5 minutes to increase blood flow and allow oil to penetrate your scalp.

Step #3 Rub oily hands down hair to treat your remaining hair.

For straighter hair, use a paddle brush to help distribute oils throughout your hair. For course or kinky hair, it is preferred to use your hands to prevent breakage from constant combing or brushing while distributing oils.

9 HAIR CARE REGIMEN

Your hair care regimen has everything to do with how well you can retain the hair growth you are working so hard for! Hair growth is inevitable if you don't have any health conditions interfering with your body's natural ability to grow hair. Retaining hair growth is possible only if you follow a proper hair care regimen unique to your specific type of hair.

The book, The Hair Care Regimen Manual, is a pocket guide that will help you by providing hair care techniques, growth advice, and hairstyles that will help you to care for your relaxed, transitioning, or natural hair. A quality hair care regimen is very important for flourishing healthy hair. Only healthy hair can truly reach longer lengths especially if growing your hair is a major goal of yours, so this manual will teach you how to grow your hair longer while at the same time, following techniques that reinforce the health of your hair.

This manual focuses on the hair care products that are needed to take care of your hair, step by step details on how to use each individual product, and ultimately a complete hair care regimen for each specific type of hair whether you are natural, transitioning, or relaxed!

The skills required to implementing your hair care regimen are of a minimum skill level paired with a vast array of hair knowledge so that you can understand why you have to do certain things to your hair, to maintain and encourage the health of it.

Next you will be provided exclusively with a Hair Care Regimen for Natural Hair that you can implement right now if you have natural hair and quality hair care products!

NATURAL HAIR CARE REGIMEN

(WEEK 1 / DAY 1)	(WEEK 2 / DAY 1)
*Shampoo *Leave In Moisturizer *Oil Sealant *Hair Gel (optional)	*Leave In Moisturizer *Oil Sealant *Hair Gel (optional)
(WEEK 1 / DAY 2)	(WEEK 2 / DAY 2)
(WEEK 1 / DAY 3)	(WEEK 2 / DAY 3)
(WEEK 1 / DAY 4)	(WEEK 2 / DAY 4)
*Co wash *Leave In Moisturizer *Oil Sealant *Hair Gel (optional)	*Co wash *Leave In Moisturizer *Oil Sealant *Hair Gel (optional)
(WEEK 1 / DAY 5)	(WEEK 2 / DAY 5)
(WEEK 1 / DAY 6)	(WEEK 2 / DAY 6)
(WEEK 1 / DAY 7) *Leave In Moisturizer	(WEEK 1 / DAY 7) *Leave In Moisturizer

Deep Condition Once A Month
Protein Treat Once A Month (If Necessary)

Feel free to moisturize more frequently if necessary

AFTERWORDS

"This manual was made for those individuals who want to do everything possible to grow their hair longer by dieting for hair growth. This manual promotes healthy eating habits and as long as you are eating an adequate supply of suggested foods high in ingredients that actually grow your hair, you will soon see great results with your growing efforts!

To preview, you have learned so much about hair beginning first with the Hair Growth Cycle to know how long it will actually take to see your growth results. Hair grows on average 1/2 an inch a month and eating for hair growth will keep you on an average track of hair growth or encourage more growth! Many who eat healthy and consume vitamins known to grow your hair, have been able to increase growth up to an inch a month! Results vary of course for each individual and with the incorporation of the advice given in this book and from consulting with your doctor, you will see a significant amount of hair growth!

Personally, I eat healthy to have a healthy body and sharper mind and my healthy thriving hair (couple with a Hair Care Regimen) is a beautiful byproduct of doing so! I notice that my hair grows a little bit faster when I consume a lot of eggs and tuna but I would rather eat a more balanced diet for my own happiness! Eating a balanced healthy diet or only eating the specific foods for hair growth is ultimately your choice because either way, you will encourage healthy hair growth so experiment with both routes to see what is best for you!

I hope that you have thoroughly enjoyed this read, it was a pleasure of mine to write this for your knowledge and enjoyment." Sincerely, Breanna

ADDITIONAL RESOURCES

The Official Website: www.Howtoblackhair.com

The Online Store: www.HowtoblackhairStore.com

Free Subscription Email: http://eepurl.com/FZs5b

For Additional Hair Questions

YourHairQuestions@Gmail.com

Black Hair Styling Tutorials

BlackWomenHair YouTube Channel

www.Youtube.com/BlackWomenHair

HowToBlackHair YouTube Channel

www.Youtube.com/HowToBlackHair

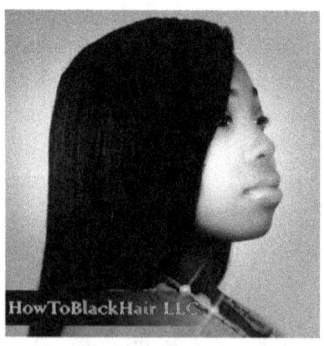

The Natural Hair Bible

The 10 Commandments of Black Hair Care

www.HowToBlackHair.com

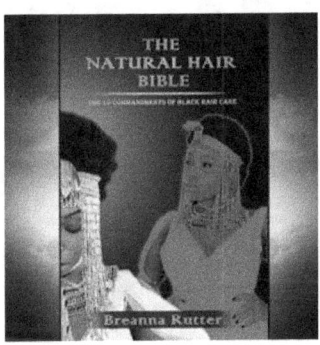

The Relaxed Hair Bible

The 10 Commandments of Long Healthy Relaxed Hair

www.HowToBlackHair.com

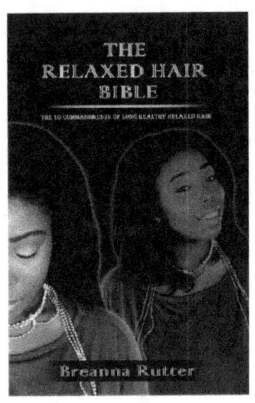

Black Hair Styling DVDs (Over 20+ Hairstyles)

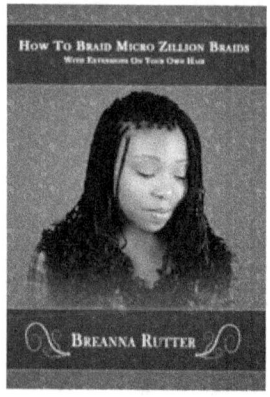 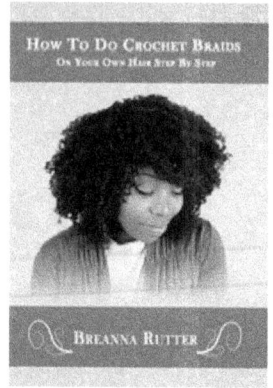

DEFINITION GUIDE

Acidic Foods: *foods that raise the acidity of your blood*
Alkaline Foods: *foods that normalize or lower the acidity of your blood*
Anagen: *the growth phase of the hair cycle*
Areata Alopecia: *hair loss cause by a reaction from your immune system*
Catagen: *the transitioning phase of the hair cycle*
Course Hair: *your individual strands of hair are the same size or bigger in size (diameter) to regular sewing thread*
Cuticles: *a naturally protecting shield (arranged like shingles to the roof of a home) outside of your hair strands*
Dermal Papilla: *a raised dermis located underneath the root of your follicle that houses the blood supply*
DHT (Dihydrotestosterone): *an enzyme that becomes from the conversion of testosterone and Type II 5-alpha reductase located in the oil gland of your hair follicle*
Elasticity: *the stretching ability of your hair*
Follicle: *an individual strand of hair*
Fine Hair: *your individual strands of hair are smaller in size (diameter) to regular sewing thread*
FUE Hair Transplant: *Follicular Unit Extraction*
FUT Hair Transplant: *Follicular Unit Transplant*
Hair Life Cycle: *the cycle of hair growth*
Hair Shaft: *a visible strand of hair*
PH Balance: *hair balanced with a PH of 4.5 to 5.5*
Sebaceous Gland: *an oil gland located underneath your scalp near the base of your hair shaft that secretes a natural oil called sebum*
Sebum: *a natural oil that protects your hair and scalp*
Shedding: *natural hair loss experienced from the catagen to telogen phase*
Telogen: *the rest phase of the hair cycle*
Thick Hair: *your ponytail width, with all of your hair gathered, is the width of a quarter or larger*
Thin Hair: *your ponytail width, with all of your hair gathered, is the width of a nickel or smaller*
Traction Alopecia: *hair loss caused by inappropriate styling or hair care practices*

HOW TO BLACK HAIR LLC.
WRITTEN BY BREANNA RUTTER
BOOK DESIGNED BY BREANNA RUTTER
COVER DESIGNED BY JARED RUTTER
ALL RIGHTS RESERVED.
VISIT WWW.HOWTOBLACKHAIR.COM

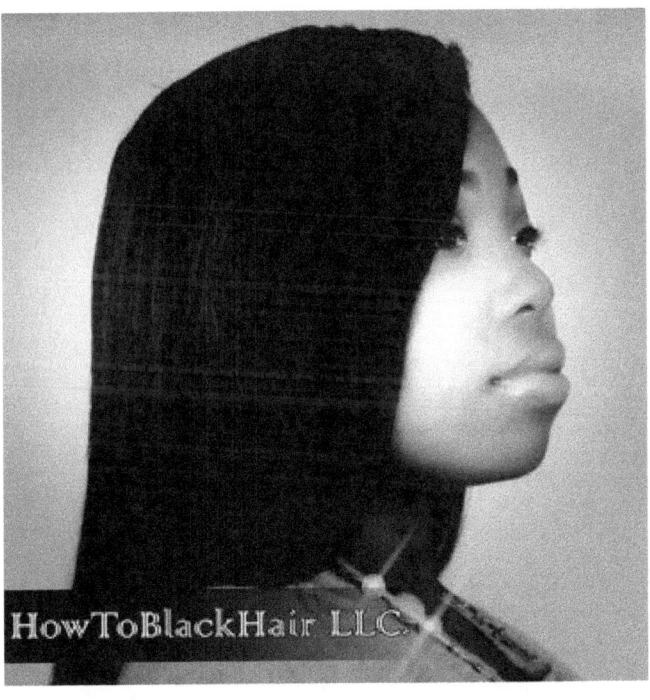

DISCLAIMER: All suggestions, techniques & advice given are for informational purposes only & should be used at your discretion & best judgment. I highly recommend conducting strand tests when trying or using new products, hair appliances & product mixes. I am not responsible or liable for adverse or undesirable affects including hair loss, hair breakage or other hair/scalp/skin/body damage as a direct or indirect result of the suggestions, tips, techniques &/or advice given.